Taming
The
Storm
Within

How to get rid of Stressed belly

CLAUDIA T. ALVES

Taming the Storm Within

How to get rid of Stressed belly

Claudia T. Alves

To my Wonderful sister Sophia

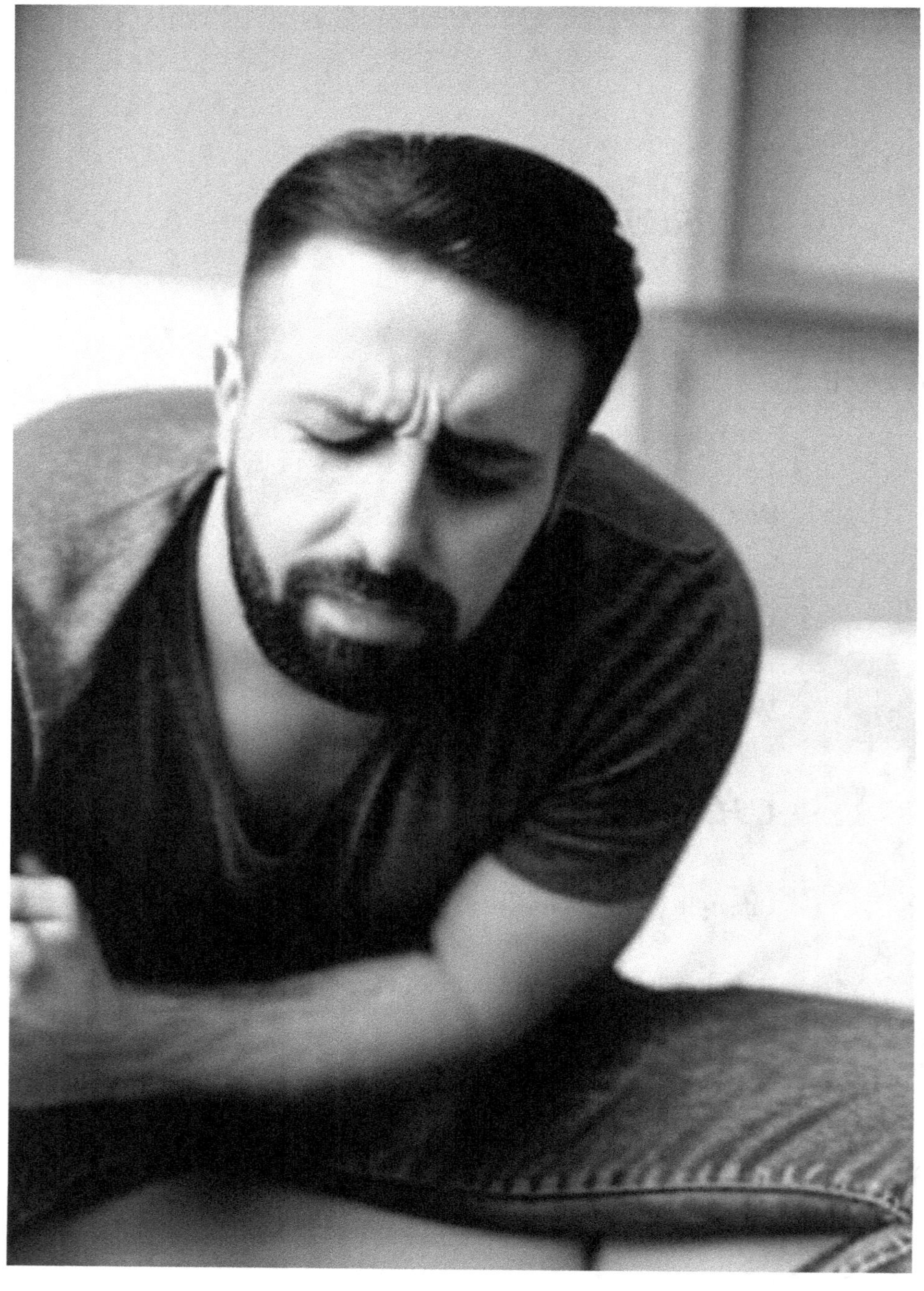

Introduction

Aitlyn had always been an ambitious person, with a drive to succeed in all aspects of her life. She was a high achiever, always striving to do better and accomplish more. She was also a workaholic, spending long hours at the office and taking on more responsibilities than she could handle. She prided herself on her ability to handle stress and push through difficult situations, but her body was beginning to show the signs of chronic stress.

Kaitlyn had gained weight, particularly around her belly, and had started to feel tired and run down all the time. She visited her doctor, who confirmed that her cortisol levels were elevated, indicating that she was under chronic stress. Kaitlyn was shocked and dismayed by the news, and she realized that she needed to take action to tame the storm within.

Just when she was researching about her condition online, she came across a blog online where she saw this book. she began to make changes to her lifestyle, starting with her diet. She cut back on sugar and processed foods, and began to eat a healthy, balanced diet with plenty of fresh fruits and vegetables. She also started to exercise regularly, going for walks or runs in the park, taking up yoga, and swimming.

Kaitlyn knew that she needed to manage her stress levels, so she started to practice mindfulness and meditation. She learned breathing techniques to help her relax and focus, and she made time for self-care and relaxation. She also started to prioritize sleep, ensuring that she got at least 7-8 hours of sleep each night. As she made these changes, Kaitlyn started to feel better and more energized. Her body began to respond positively, and she started to lose weight, particularly around her belly. She felt happier, more relaxed, and more in control of her life.

Kaitlyn also began to explore natural supplements and herbs to help her manage her stress levels. She started taking probiotics to improve her gut health, which has been linked to reduced stress levels. She also tried adaptogenic herbs like ashwagandha and rhodiola, which are known to reduce cortisol levels and promote relaxation.

Over time, Kaitlyn learned to listen to her body and prioritize her own well-being. She realized that taking care of herself was the key to achieving success in all areas of her life. She continued to make small, positive changes to her lifestyle, and these changes added up over time.

Today, Kaitlyn is a successful businesswoman, but she no longer sacrifices her health and well-being for her career. She has tamed the storm within, and she feels happier, healthier, and more fulfilled than ever before.

Stressed belly

I'm sure you all know what's stress is all about so let's skip to the point.

Stressed belly, also known as stress belly or cortisol belly, refers to the accumulation of fat in the abdominal area due to chronic stress. The hormone cortisol, which is released by the adrenal glands in response to stress, is a main contributor to stressed belly. Cortisol stimulates the body to store fat in the abdominal area, as this was once an evolutionary advantage for survival during periods of stress or famine.

Stressed belly can also be caused by a combination of factors including poor diet, lack of exercise, lack of sleep, and medical conditions.

It is important to address stressed belly not only for aesthetic reasons, but also for overall health as this type of fat is associated with increased risk for several health problems such as heart disease, diabetes, and high blood pressure.

Lifestyle changes such as exercise, healthy eating, stress management techniques, and getting enough sleep can help to reduce stress and decrease the amount of belly fat. Additionally, supplements and herbs such as probiotics, adaptogenic herbs, and essential oils can also be helpful in reducing stress levels and belly fat. In severe cases, medical intervention may be necessary.

Taming the storm within refers to managing and reducing chronic stress, which can have a significant impact on our health and well-being.

Chronic stress can lead to the release of the hormone cortisol, which in turn can lead to the accumulation of belly fat, also known as stressed belly. Stressed belly is associated with increased health risks such as heart disease, diabetes, and high blood pressure.

Taming the storm within is important for overall health and

preventing the negative effects of chronic stress. By managing stress through lifestyle changes such as exercise, healthy eating, stress management techniques, and getting enough sleep, we can reduce the amount of cortisol in our bodies and decrease the amount of belly fat.

In addition to physical health benefits, managing stress through taming the storm within can also improve our emotional and mental well-being, leading to increased happiness, better relationships, and a more fulfilling life.

Therefore, taming the storm within is a crucial step towards a healthier, happier, and more balanced life.

Chapter 1

The relationship between stress and belly fat

The connection between stress and belly fat is a complex and well-established phenomenon. Chronic stress can lead to the release of the hormone cortisol, which can have a significant impact on the accumulation of fat in the abdominal area, commonly referred to as stressed belly.

When the body experiences stress, the adrenal glands release cortisol, which is a stress hormone. Cortisol signals the body to release glucose, a source of energy, into the bloodstream. It also signals the body to store fat in the abdominal area, as this was once an evolutionary advantage for survival during periods of stress or famine.

However, in today's world, where stress is a constant presence in many people's lives, the constant release of cortisol can lead to an accumulation of fat in the abdominal area. This type of fat, known as stressed belly fat, is particularly concerning because it is associated with increased health risks such as heart disease, diabetes, and high blood pressure.

The science behind stressed belly is rooted in the concept of insulin resistance. When cortisol levels are elevated, they can increase insulin resistance, leading to higher insulin levels and an increased risk of belly fat. This is because insulin stimulates fat storage, and elevated insulin levels can lead to the accumulation of fat in the abdominal area.

Understanding the connection between stress and belly fat is crucial for managing chronic stress and reducing the risk of health problems associated with stressed belly. By controlling cortisol levels through lifestyle changes such as exercise, healthy eating, stress management techniques, and getting enough sleep, individuals can reduce their risk of developing stressed belly and improve their overall health and well-being

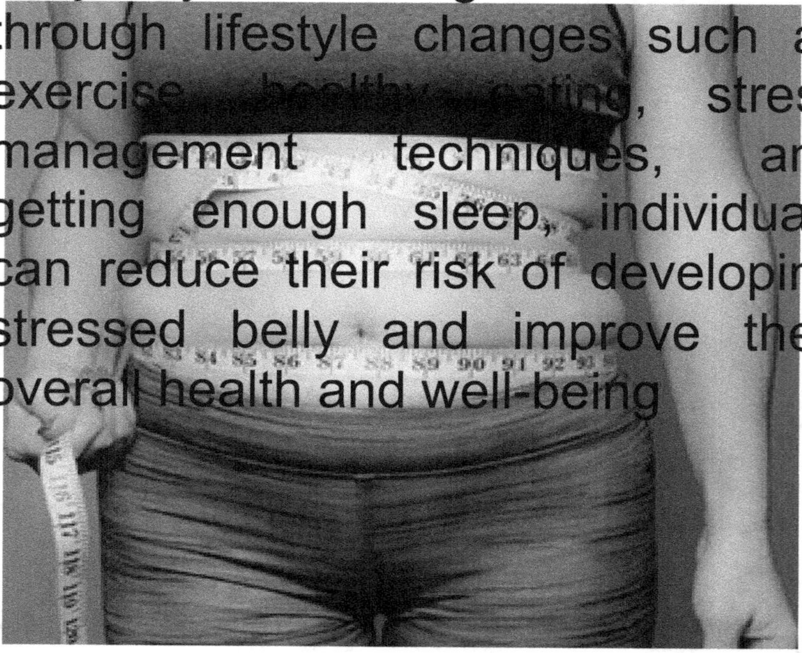

How stress affects the body

Stress has a profound impact on the body, and understanding how stress affects the body is essential for managing chronic stress and reducing its negative effects. Here are some key points on how stress affects the body:

❖ Cortisol release: Stress triggers the release of cortisol, a hormone produced by the adrenal glands that regulates metabolism, immune function, and blood pressure. Cortisol levels are naturally higher in the morning and lower at night, but chronic stress can result in elevated cortisol levels throughout the day.

❖ Increased heart rate: Stress can also increase the heart rate and blood pressure, which can put additional strain on the heart and cardiovascular system.

❖ Suppressed immune system: Cortisol has a suppressive effect on the immune system, which can lead to an increased risk of infection and illness.

- ❖ Digestive issues: Stress can also affect digestion, leading to symptoms such as acid reflux, stomach cramps, and diarrhea.
- ❖ Mental and emotional effects: Chronic stress can also impact mental and emotional health, leading to symptoms such as anxiety, depression, and irritability.

Did You Know?

"In women, Stress may mess up your regular menstrual cycles"

Chapter 2

What really causes Stressed belly

The science behind stressed belly is rooted in the connection between stress, cortisol levels, and insulin resistance. Stress triggers the release of cortisol, a hormone produced by the adrenal glands that regulates metabolism, immune function, and blood pressure. Cortisol levels are naturally higher in the morning and lower at night, but chronic stress can result in elevated cortisol levels throughout the day.

This can lead to insulin resistance and an increased risk of belly fat.

Cortisol is a hormone produced by the adrenal glands in response to stress, and it plays a critical role in the development of stressed belly. Here are some key points on the role of cortisol in stressed belly:

❖ Regulates metabolism: Cortisol regulates metabolism by stimulating the release of glucose, a source of energy, into the bloodstream. It also helps to regulate blood pressure and immune function.

❖ Insulin resistance: Chronic stress and elevated cortisol levels can increase insulin resistance, leading to higher insulin levels and an increased risk of belly fat. This is because insulin stimulates fat storage, and elevated insulin levels can lead to the accumulation of fat in the abdominal area.

❖ Suppresses immune system: Cortisol has a suppressive effect on the immune system, which can lead to an increased risk of infection and illness.

❖ Increased heart rate: Stress can also increase the heart rate and blood pressure, which can put additional strain on the heart and cardiovascular system.

❖ Mental and emotional effects: Chronic stress can also impact mental and emotional health, leading to symptoms such as anxiety, depression, and irritability.

cortisol is a key player in the development of stressed belly and its associated health risks. By reducing cortisol levels through lifestyle changes such as exercise, healthy eating, stress management techniques, and getting enough sleep, individuals can mitigate the impact of stress on their bodies and overall health.

Cortisol and insulin work together to regulate glucose levels in the bloodstream. Cortisol signals the body to release glucose, a source of energy, into the bloodstream, while insulin regulates the uptake of glucose into cells. When cortisol levels are elevated, they can increase insulin resistance, leading to higher insulin levels and an increased risk of belly fat. This is because insulin stimulates fat storage, and elevated insulin levels can lead to the accumulation of fat in the abdominal area.

Chronic stress is another common cause of stressed belly and the accumulation of belly fat. Chronic stress can be caused by a variety of day-to-day activities, including:

❖ Work-related stress: Long hours, heavy workloads, tight deadlines, and demanding bosses can all contribute to chronic stress.

❖ Financial stress: Money worries, such as paying bills or making ends meet, can also lead to chronic stress.

❖ Relationship stress: Struggles in personal relationships, whether with partners, family members, or friends, can cause chronic stress.

❖ Health-related stress: Chronic health problems, such as chronic pain, can also contribute to chronic stress.

❖ Caregiving stress: Caring for a loved one, such as an elderly parent or a child with special needs, can also cause chronic stress.

❖ Commuting stress: Daily commutes, especially in congested areas, can also contribute to chronic stress.

❖ Technology-related stress: Constantly being connected to technology, such as emails and social media, can also lead to chronic stress. Here are some key points on chronic stress as a cause of stressed belly:

❖ Elevated cortisol levels: Chronic stress triggers the release of cortisol, a hormone that regulates metabolism, immune function, and blood pressure. When cortisol levels are elevated, they can increase insulin resistance and lead to an increased risk of belly fat.

❖ Poor eating habits: Chronic stress can also lead to unhealthy eating habits, such as overeating or consuming sugary and fatty foods. This can contribute to an increased risk of belly fat and overall weight gain.

❖ Lack of physical activity: Chronic stress can also reduce physical activity, leading to a sedentary lifestyle and decreased calorie expenditure.

❖ Sleep deprivation: Chronic stress can also impact sleep quality, leading to sleep deprivation and elevated cortisol levels.

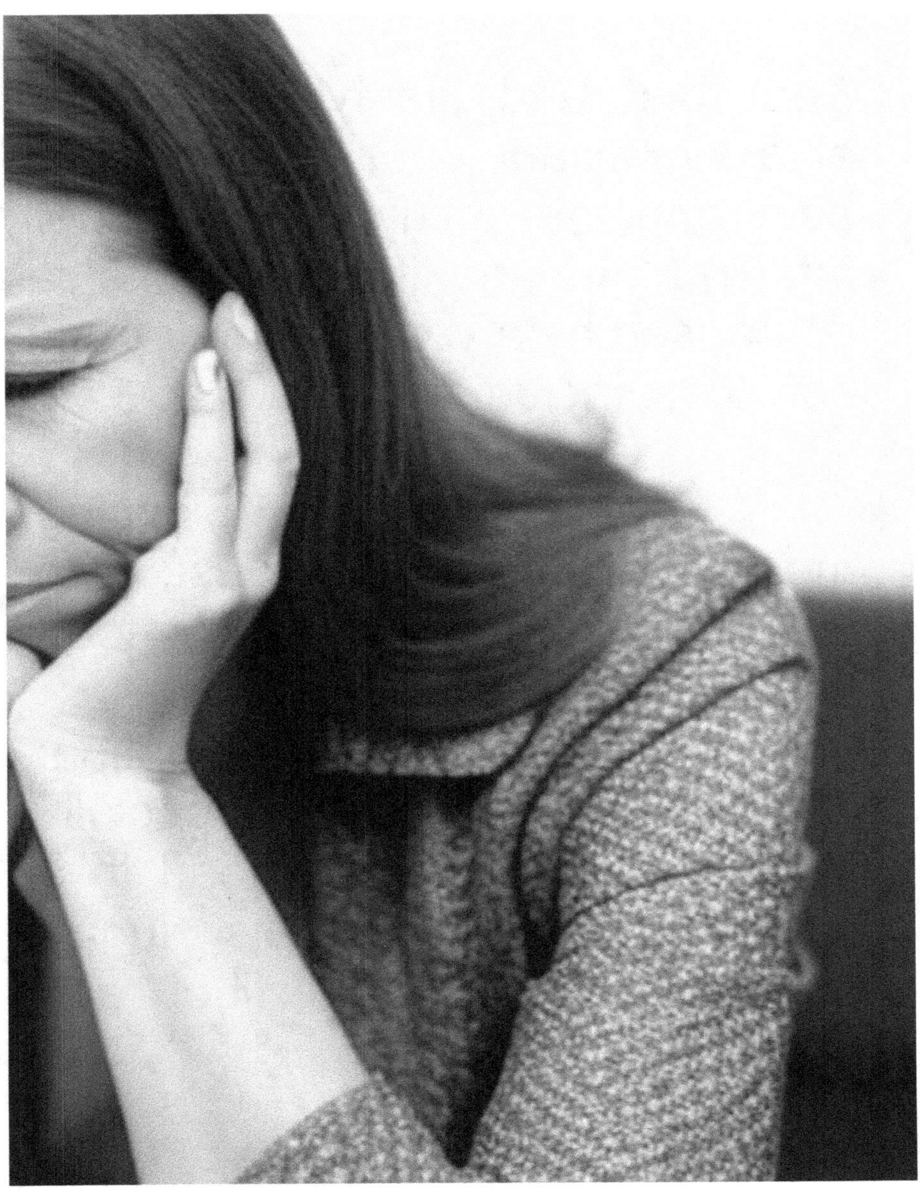

Poor diet and lifestyle habits are also significant causes of stressed belly and the accumulation of belly fat. Poor diet and lifestyle habits can be caused by a variety of day-to-day activities, including:

❖ Skipping meals: Skipping meals, especially breakfast, can lead to overeating and poor food choices later in the day.

❖ Fast food consumption: Consuming fast food, especially on a regular basis, can lead to a diet high in unhealthy fats, sugar, and salt, and low in fiber and nutrients.

❖   Lack of physical activity: A sedentary lifestyle, such as sitting for long periods at work or in front of the TV, can lead to decreased calorie expenditure and a higher risk of weight gain.

❖Poor sleep habits: Lack of sleep, or poor sleep quality, can disrupt hormones and metabolism, leading to weight gain and poor diet choices.

❖Smoking: Smoking can disrupt hunger hormones and metabolism, leading to weight gain and poor diet choices.

❖Excessive alcohol consumption: Excessive alcohol consumption can contribute to a high-calorie diet and decreased physical activity levels. Here are some key points on the role of poor diet and lifestyle in the development of stressed belly:

❖ High sugar and processed food intake: A diet high in sugar and processed foods can lead to insulin resistance and elevated cortisol levels, contributing to the accumulation of belly fat.

❖ Lack of fiber and nutrient-rich foods: A diet lacking in fiber and nutrient-rich foods can lead to digestive problems and increased inflammation, both of which can contribute to stressed belly.

❖ Sedentary lifestyle: A sedentary lifestyle can lead to decreased calorie expenditure, which can contribute to weight gain and the accumulation of belly fat.

❖ Lack of physical activity: Lack of physical activity can also lead to decreased muscle mass and a slower metabolism, both of which can contribute to weight gain and stressed belly.

❖ Smoking and excessive alcohol consumption: Smoking and excessive alcohol consumption can also impact health, leading to increased inflammation, oxidative stress, and elevated cortisol levels.

Medical conditions can also contribute to stressed belly and the accumulation of belly fat. Medical conditions can be caused by a variety of day-to-day activities, including:

❖ Poor diet and lifestyle habits: A diet high in unhealthy fats, sugar, and salt, and low in fiber and nutrients, combined with a sedentary lifestyle, can increase the risk of developing medical conditions such as type 2 diabetes, heart disease, and certain cancers.

- ❖ Smoking: Smoking can increase the risk of developing a range of medical conditions, including heart disease, stroke, and lung cancer.
- ❖ Excessive alcohol consumption: Excessive alcohol consumption can increase the risk of liver disease, pancreatitis, and certain cancers.
- ❖ Lack of physical activity: A sedentary lifestyle can increase the risk of developing a range of medical conditions, including heart disease, type 2 diabetes, and certain cancers.

- ❖ Stress: Chronic stress can increase the risk of developing medical conditions such as cardiovascular disease, depression, and anxiety.

- ❖ Environmental exposure: Exposure to environmental pollutants, such as air pollution and toxic chemicals, can increase the risk of developing medical conditions such as respiratory problems, certain cancers, and neurological disorders. Here are some key points on the role of medical conditions in the development of stressed belly:

- ❖ Hormonal imbalances: Hormonal imbalances, such as those seen in conditions such as polycystic ovary syndrome (PCOS) and thyroid disorders, can contribute to the accumulation of belly fat.
- ❖ Inflammatory conditions: Chronic inflammatory conditions, such as arthritis and Crohn's disease, can also contribute to stressed belly and an increased risk of belly fat.
- ❖ Metabolic disorders: Metabolic disorders, such as type 2 diabetes, can also increase the risk of belly fat due to elevated insulin levels and insulin resistance.

❖ Medications: Certain medications, such as steroids and some antidepressants, can increase the risk of belly fat and contribute to stressed belly.

Stressed belly fat is particularly concerning because it is associated with increased health risks such as heart disease, diabetes, and high blood pressure. This type of fat, known as visceral fat, is stored deep within the abdomen, surrounding the organs. Unlike subcutaneous fat, which is stored just below the skin, visceral fat is metabolically active, producing hormones and cytokines that can affect health.

Studies have shown that individuals with higher levels of belly fat are at an increased risk of developing insulin resistance and type 2 diabetes, as well as cardiovascular disease and certain types of cancer. This is because stressed belly fat produces hormones and cytokines that can increase inflammation, oxidative stress, and insulin resistance, leading to an increased risk of chronic diseases.

Chapter 3

Lifestyle Changes to Reduce cortisol level

Lifestyle changes can have a significant impact on reducing stressed belly and managing cortisol levels.

Lifestyle changes can play an important role in taming the storm within and reducing the risk of developing stressed belly.

Regular exercise is an effective way to reduce cortisol levels, as it helps to reduce stress and improve insulin sensitivity. Exercise can also help to increase muscle mass, which can help to reduce belly fat. Regular exercise and physical activity can play a crucial role in reducing the risk of developing stressed belly. Physical activity can help reduce cortisol levels and improve the body's stress response, which can help reduce the risk of developing stressed belly. Exercise can also help improve insulin sensitivity and promote weight loss, which can further help reduce the risk of developing stressed belly.

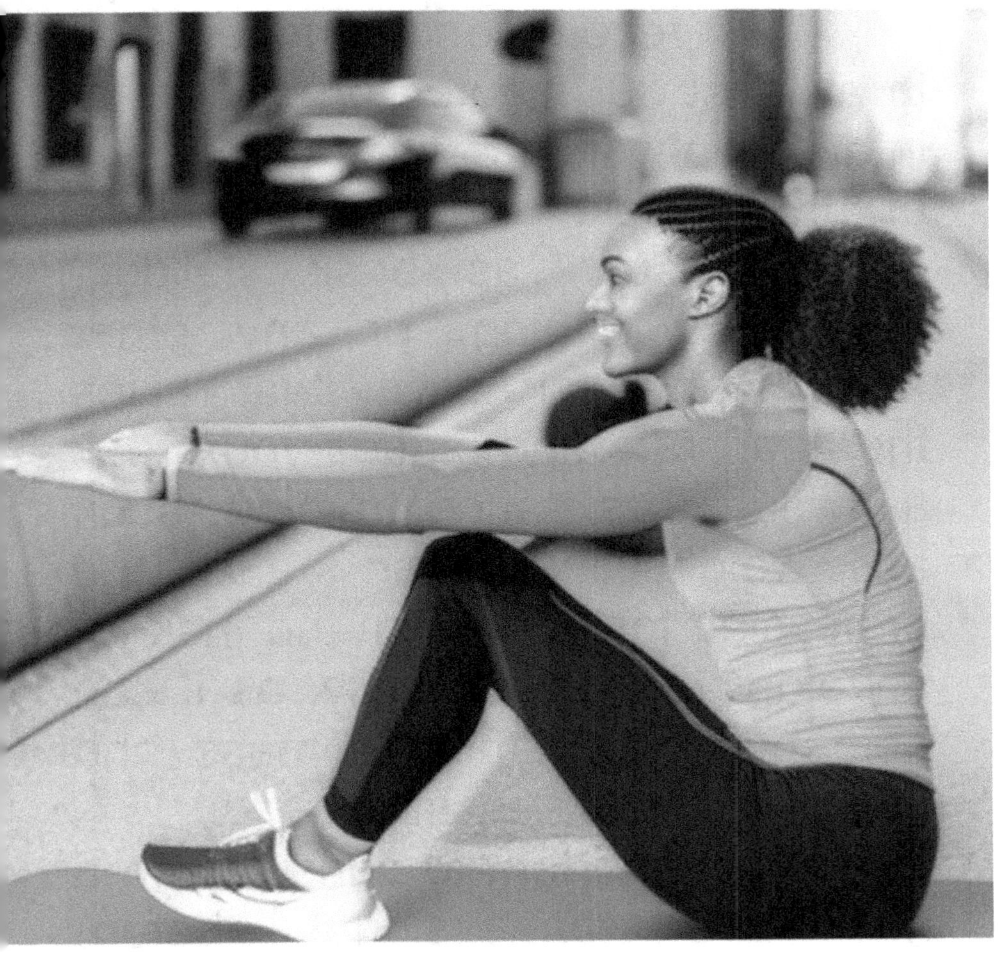

It is recommended to engage in at least 30 minutes of moderate-intensity physical activity most days of the week. This can include activities such as brisk walking, cycling, swimming, or any other form of physical activity that raises the heart rate and makes you break a sweat. Resistance training, such as weightlifting, can also be beneficial for reducing the risk of developing stressed belly, as it can help build lean muscle mass and improve insulin sensitivity.

It is important to consult with a healthcare professional before starting a new exercise regimen, especially if you have any underlying medical conditions or have been inactive for an extended period of time. A healthcare professional can help you determine the best type and intensity of exercise for your individual needs and goals.

Mindfulness and meditation practices, such as yoga and tai chi, can also help to reduce cortisol levels and manage stress. These practices can help to calm the mind and body, reduce anxiety, and improve overall well-being. They are techniques that involve focusing the mind on the present moment and quieting the inner dialogue. These techniques have been shown to have a number of benefits for reducing stress and improving overall health and well-being, including reducing cortisol levels and improving the body's stress response.

Research has shown that mindfulness and meditation can help reduce symptoms of stress, anxiety, and depression, which can contribute to the development of stressed belly. Regular practice of mindfulness and meditation can help promote relaxation, reduce negative thoughts and emotions, and improve overall mental and emotional well-being.

There are a number of mindfulness and meditation techniques that can be practiced, including deep breathing, guided imagery, and body scans. It is recommended to start with a simple technique and gradually build up to more advanced practices as you become more comfortable with the practice.

It is important to note that mindfulness and meditation should not be used as a substitute for other forms of treatment, such as therapy or medication, if needed. It is always best to consult with a healthcare professional to determine the best course of treatment for your individual needs and goals.

Getting enough sleep is a crucial for managing cortisol levels. Getting quality sleep are crucial components of reducing the risk of developing stressed belly. Sleep and stress management techniques can help reduce cortisol levels and improve the body's stress response, which can help reduce the risk of developing stressed belly, as sleep deprivation can result in elevated cortisol levels. Aiming for 7-9 hours of quality sleep each night can help to reduce cortisol levels and improve insulin sensitivity.

In some cases, therapy or medication may be necessary to effectively manage stress, and a healthcare professional can help determine the best course of treatment for your individual needs and goals.

Healthy eating habits, such as reducing sugar and processed foods, can also help to reduce cortisol levels and reduce the risk of belly fat. Eating a diet that is rich in fiber, lean protein, and healthy fats can help to reduce inflammation, regulate glucose levels, and improve insulin sensitivity.

A healthy diet is an important aspect of reducing the risk of developing stressed belly. Eating a diet that is rich in fiber, lean protein, healthy fats, and complex carbohydrates can help reduce cortisol levels and improve the body's stress response.

It is recommended to limit the intake of sugar and processed foods, as these foods have been linked to higher cortisol levels and an increased risk of stressed belly. Additionally, consuming a diet that is rich in fruits, vegetables, and whole grains can help reduce the risk of developing stressed belly, as these foods are rich in nutrients that support overall health and well-being.

Drinking plenty of water and limiting the intake of caffeine and alcohol can also help reduce cortisol levels and improve the body's stress response. Caffeine and alcohol are stimulants that can disrupt sleep and increase cortisol levels, which can contribute to the development of stressed belly.

Did you Know?

"Chronic stress can cause substance abuse"

Chapter 4

How to get rid of stress belly Fat

The importance of exercise

The key to total health and well-being is exercise. Frequent exercise helps strengthen the immune system, lower blood pressure, and lower the risk of developing chronic conditions including type 2 diabetes and some malignancies. Exercise releases endorphins, the body's natural mood boosters, which can help manage stress and increase mood.

Exercise has many health advantages for the body, but it can also enhance memory and cognitive performance. Regular exercise has been demonstrated in studies to help prevent cognitive deterioration and lower the risk of Stressed belly. Moreover, exercise can enhance the quality of sleep, which is crucial for general health and well-being. So, choosing an exercise regimen that you enjoy and can keep can have many advantages for your physical and mental health, whether it's a daily stroll, a yoga class, or a weightlifting session.

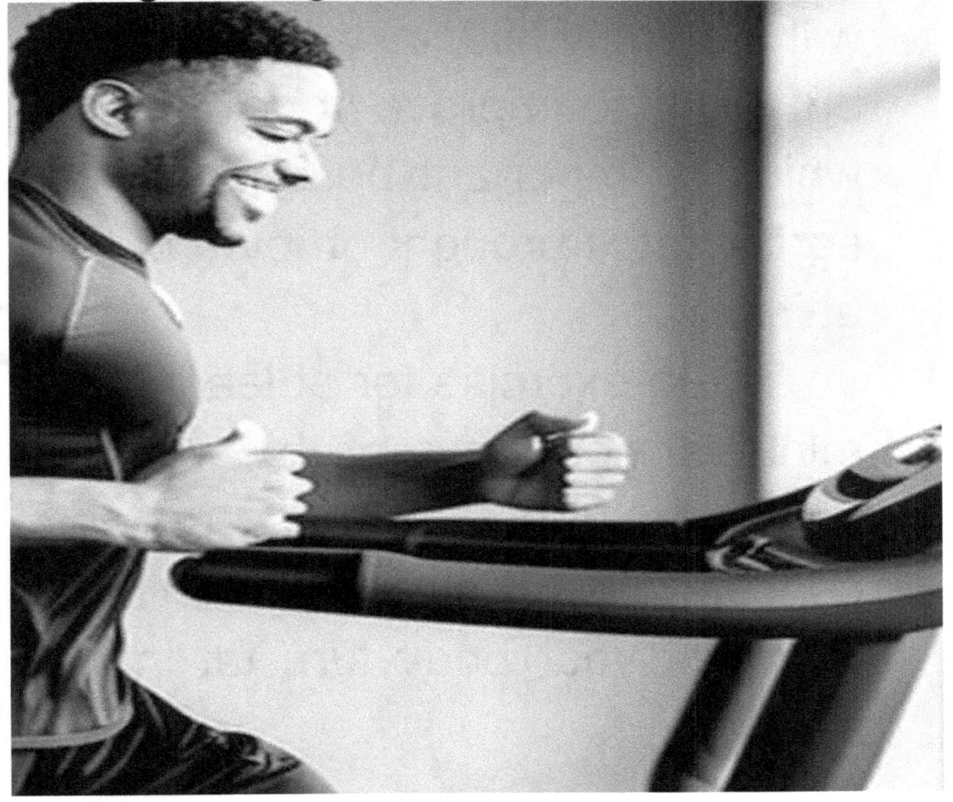

You must exercise and keep a calorie deficit to lose stress belly fat, just like it is with any other sort of body fat. Exercise will not only aid in weight loss but will also improve your mood, which is important because this sort of fat is brought on by a bad attitude

Try to exercise for at least 30 minutes most days of the week, and on the other days, concentrate on strength training to assist your body turn fat into muscle.

Consume more high-fiber foods.

An often-overlooked yet crucial part of a balanced diet is fiber. A diet high in fiber has many advantages, such as improving digestion, encouraging regularity, lowering the risk of certain illnesses like heart disease, and assisting with weight management.

Fiber is well known for helping with digestion. Everyone who is stressed should consider adding it to their diet because of this. This is because indigestion and constipation are common digestive issues for those who are under stress. These problems can be resolved by consuming more fiber-rich foods including beans, chia seeds, and bran cereal.

Fruits, vegetables, whole grains, legumes, nuts, and seeds are among the foods high in fiber. Adults should consume at least 25 to 30 grams of fiber daily, however, many people fall short of this recommendation. Include a variety of fiber-rich foods in your diet, and choose whole foods rather than heavily processed ones, to improve your consumption of fiber.

Starting the day with a high-fiber breakfast like oatmeal, whole-wheat bread, or a fruit smoothie with additional chia or flax seeds is one approach to improve fiber consumption. Choose fruit, nuts, seeds, or raw vegetables with hummus as your snack options. Focus on filling your plate with extra fruits and veggies and nutritious grains like quinoa, brown rice, or whole-grain pasta. In addition to being great sources of fiber, legumes like lentils, chickpeas, and black beans can also be used in soups, stews, and salads. You may improve your fiber intake and reap the many health advantages of a fiber-rich diet by making little dietary modifications.

Observe what you eat.

Maintaining a healthy lifestyle involves many different factors, including watching what you eat. It is critical to pay attention to the type and amount of food that you eat every day. Your body can acquire the nutrients it requires to function at its best by consuming a balanced diet that consists of a variety of nutrient-dense foods like fruits, vegetables, whole grains, lean proteins, and healthy fats. The risk of chronic diseases like obesity, type 2 diabetes, and heart disease can be increased by consuming a lot of highly processed meals, sugary drinks, and foods high in saturated and trans fats.

Making a grocery list and sticking to it can help you control what you eat by helping you plan your meals ahead of time. Shop without being hungry because doing so can result in impulsive purchases of harmful items. By paying attention to your body's hunger and fullness cues, portion control and mindful eating are also beneficial. You can learn to tune in to your body's signals by eating slowly, chewing your meal carefully, and avoiding distractions like devices while you're eating. Your general health and wellness can be enhanced by adopting minor dietary adjustments and eating with awareness. Take a quick survey to receive a meal and exercise plan.

Bathing in a hot tub

Lowering cortisol levels in the body can be accomplished by taking a hot bath. Also, taking a bath raises your body temperature, which raises endorphin levels in the brain, which instantly improves your mood.

Many advantages for both physical and mental health might result from taking regular hot baths. The warmth of the water helps ease aches and pains by relaxing the muscles and lowering tension. Moreover, taking hot baths can assist to increase circulation, reducing blood pressure, and enhance skin health. A hot bath can also have a relaxing impact on the mind and lower levels of stress and anxiety. By assisting the body in relaxing and preparing for sleep, it can also encourage better sleep.

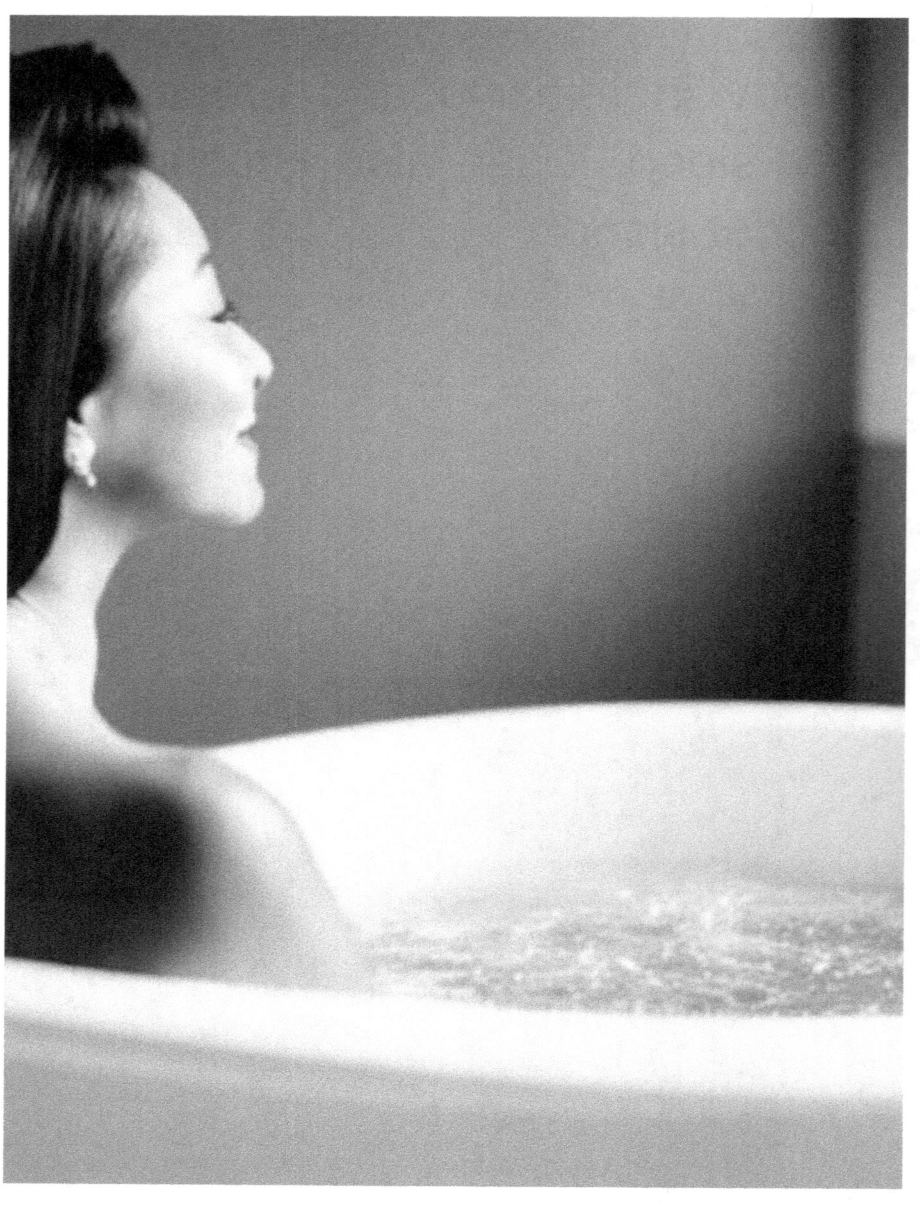

It's crucial to take the proper precautions when having a hot bath to prevent overheating or dehydration. It is advised to keep the water temperature between 37 and 39 °C (98 and 102 °F) and to keep the bath time to 20 to 30 minutes. Drinking water before and after the bath will help you keep hydrated. Epsom salts, aromatic oils, or other bath products can be used to increase the bath's medicinal and calming effects. All things considered, regular hot bathing can be a quick and efficient strategy to enhance both physical and mental well-being.

So here are some other ways to get rid of stressed belly

- Eat nutrient-dense meals.
- Go on a stroll daily, and make at least 10,000 steps each day.
- Develop more muscle by partaking in more weight and resistance training than cardio.

- Consume more protein.
- Obtain more sunlight.
- Eat more fiber-rich foods.
- Obtain a decent night's sleep, and establish a consistent sleep habit.
- Avoid smoking.
- Minimize alcohol intake.
- Eat a balanced diet rich in fruits, vegetables, and whole grains.
- Workout every day.
- Minimize stress and learn how to healthily handle stress.

Chapter 5

How to prevent stress belly

If you don't have stress belly and wish to minimize your chance for having the condition:

o   Find strategies to decrease and manage with stress: It can be taking your dog for a walk or listening to music just do what helps you to relax the most in order to reduce your stress level

- o manage your diet: Eating foods for their healthy benefits not just for cravings can help a long way to prevent one from having a stressed belly. So watch what you take

- o maintain a balanced diet: Maintaining an healthy diet is a crucial step in avoiding stressed belly

- o start exercising a little every day: Just do that exercise. Even tho you are a workaholic and don't have time, try to create a little time for an exercise everyday.

o   Don't continue to smoke or quit smoking if you presently do. If you smoke and you want to do away with getting stressed belly you have to stop smoking once and for all

o   drink alcohol moderately: Learn to do without alcohol as this leads to the accumulation of fat in the stomach.

Using Supplements and herbs
to reverse stressed belly

Supplements and herbs can play a role in reducing the risk of developing stressed belly. One such supplement is probiotics.

Probiotics: Probiotics are live bacteria and yeast that can help improve digestive health by restoring balance to the gut microbiome. Research suggests that probiotics may also help reduce inflammation, improve insulin sensitivity, and promote weight loss, which can help reduce the risk of developing stressed belly. Some good sources of probiotics include yogurt, kefir, sauerkraut, and kimchi.

Please note that while supplements and herbs can play a role in reducing the risk of developing stressed belly, they should not be used as a substitute for a balanced diet and healthy lifestyle. It is always best to consult with a healthcare professional before starting any new supplement regimen to ensure safety and effectiveness.

Adaptogenic Herbs: Adaptogenic herbs are plants that can help the body adapt to stress and promote overall health and well-being. Some popular adaptogenic herbs include ashwagandha, rhodiola, and ginseng. These herbs are believed to help reduce cortisol levels and improve the body's stress response, which can help reduce the risk of developing stressed belly.

Also note that while adaptogenic herbs may have potential benefits for reducing the risk of developing stressed belly, they should not be used as a substitute for a balanced diet and healthy lifestyle. It is always best to consult with a healthcare professional before starting any new supplement regimen to ensure safety and effectiveness. Additionally, some adaptogenic herbs may interact with certain medications, so it is important to be aware of potential risks and side effects.

Essential Oils: Essential oils are highly concentrated plant extracts that are used for their fragrance and therapeutic properties. Some essential oils that are commonly used for reducing stress and improving overall health and well-being include lavender, peppermint, and lemon. These oils are believed to help reduce cortisol levels and improve the body's stress response, which can help reduce the risk of developing stressed belly.

It is important to note that while essential oils may have potential benefits for reducing the risk of developing stressed belly, they should not be used as a substitute for a balanced diet and healthy lifestyle. It is always best to consult with a healthcare professional before starting any new supplement regimen to ensure safety and effectiveness. Additionally, some essential oils may interact with certain medications or cause skin irritation, so it is important to be aware of potential risks and side effects. Essential oils should always be used in dilution and never applied undiluted to the skin.

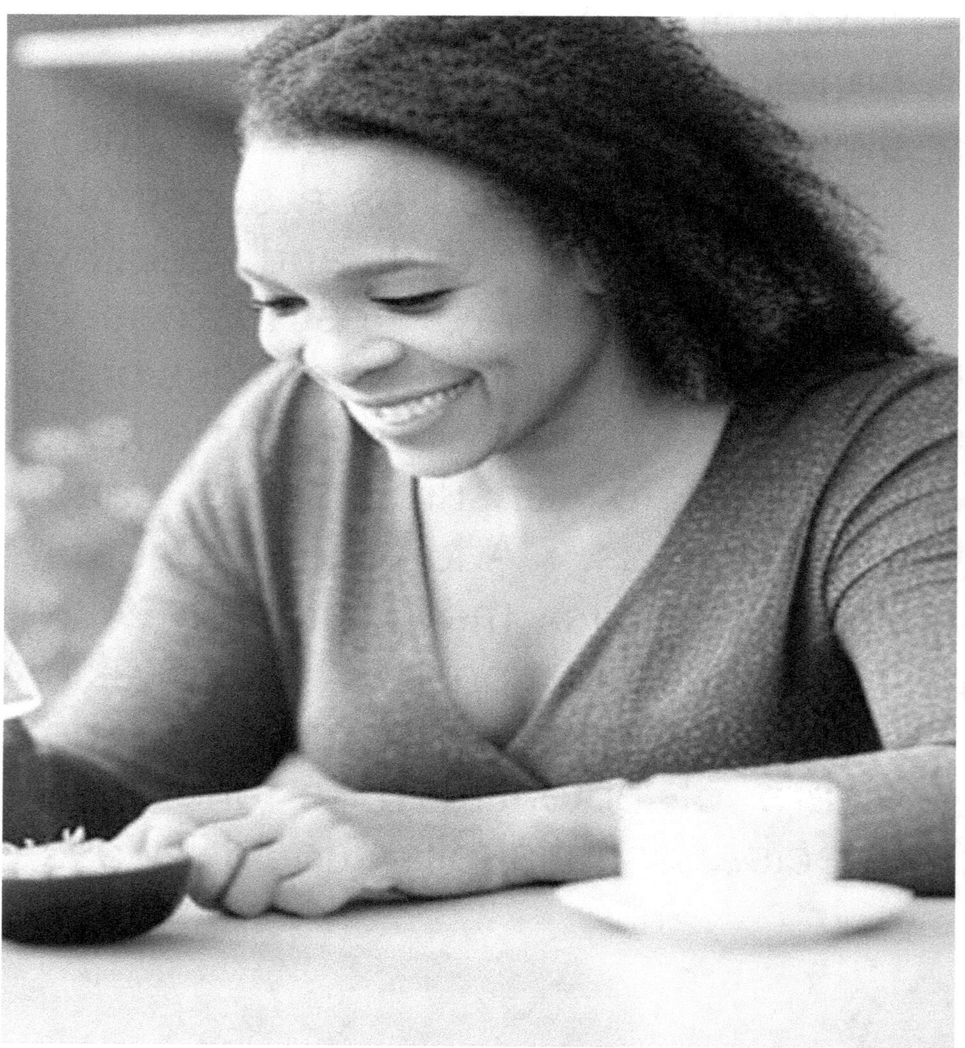

Did you Know?

"Stress increase your risk for type 2 diabetes"

Chapter 6

Medical Interventions for Stressed Belly

Medications: In some cases, medications may be necessary to effectively manage stressed belly. There are a variety of medications that may be used to treat stressed belly, including anti-anxiety medications, antidepressants, and beta blockers.

Anti-anxiety medications, such as benzodiazepines, can help reduce symptoms of anxiety and improve the body's stress response.

Antidepressants, such as selective serotonin reuptake inhibitors (SSRIs), can help regulate cortisol levels and improve the body's stress response.

Beta blockers, such as propranolol, can help reduce cortisol levels and improve the body's stress response by blocking the effects of adrenaline and reducing physical symptoms of stress, such as heart palpitations and sweating.

In some cases, therapy or lifestyle changes may be necessary to effectively manage stressed belly, and a healthcare professional can help determine the best course of treatment for your individual needs and goals.

Surgery: In severe cases of stressed belly, surgery may be necessary to effectively manage symptoms. There are a variety of surgical options that may be used to treat stressed belly, including liposuction and abdominoplasty.

Liposuction is a minimally invasive procedure that removes excess fat from the abdominal area. This procedure can be effective in reducing the appearance of stressed belly, but it is important to note that liposuction is not a weight-loss solution and should not be used as a substitute for a healthy diet and lifestyle.

Abdominoplasty, also known as a tummy tuck, is a surgical procedure that removes excess skin and fat from the abdominal area. This procedure can be effective in reducing the appearance of stressed belly, but it is important to note that abdominoplasty is a major surgery and carries associated risks and potential complications.

It is important to consult with a healthcare professional to determine the best course of treatment for your individual needs and goals. In many cases, lifestyle changes, such as exercise and healthy eating habits, may be necessary to effectively manage stressed belly, and a healthcare professional can help determine the best course of treatment for your individual needs and goals.

Other Medical Treatments: In addition to medications and surgery, there are other medical treatments that may be used to manage stressed belly. These may include:

Hormone therapy: Hormone therapy may be used to regulate cortisol levels and improve the body's stress response.

Cortisol blockers: Cortisol blockers may be used to prevent

cortisol from being produced and released in response to stress.

Fat-loss injections: Fat-loss injections, such as Lipostabil, can help reduce excess fat from the abdominal area.

Infrared light therapy: Infrared light therapy may be used to reduce inflammation and improve the body's stress response.

It is important to consult with a healthcare professional to determine the best course of treatment for your individual needs and goals. In some cases, a combination of medical treatments and lifestyle changes may be necessary to effectively manage stressed belly, and a healthcare professional can help determine the best course of treatment for your individual needs and goals.

Did you Know?

"High blood pressure develops from chronic stress"

Chapter 7

Finally to maintain a healthy lifestyle for a stress-free belly, the author suggests engaging in regular exercise and physical activity, practicing mindfulness and meditation, prioritizing adequate sleep and utilizing stress management techniques, and adopting healthy eating habits. It is also important to monitor stress levels and make changes as needed to ensure the body remains in a state of balance and wellness. This may include reducing stress in work and personal life, engaging in self-care and relaxation, and making time for physical activity and rest. By incorporating these habits into daily life, individuals can achieve a happier, healthier life free from the negative effects of stress and stressed belly.

Dear Reader,

Thank you so much for taking the time to read "Taming the Storm Within: How to Get Rid of Stressed Belly." It means a great deal to me that you have chosen to invest in your health and wellbeing by exploring the strategies and insights presented in this book.

I truly hope that you have found the information helpful, and that you have gained a deeper understanding of the gut-brain connection and the importance of managing stress for optimal health. My greatest desire is to empower you to take control of your health and wellbeing, and to provide you with practical tools that you can use to reduce stress and inflammation in your body.

If there is anything else that I can do to support you on your journey, please do not hesitate to reach out. I am grateful for your trust and your commitment to your health, and I wish you all the best on your path to wellness.

With gratitude,

Claudia